New Keto Diet: Meat and Vegan Cookbook 2021

The easiest keto recipes for everyone

Sommario

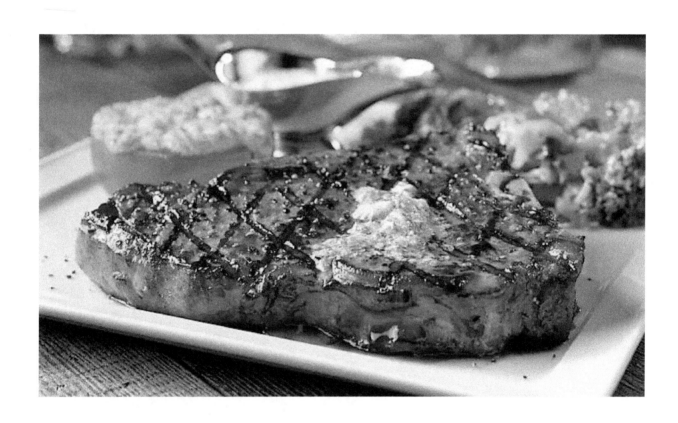

INTRODUCTION

Welcome to the wonderful world of keto meat. This book is a collection of the best meat recipes cooked and prepared keto style. As you know, meat is one of the richest sources of protein and is excellent for following the keto diet and having excellent results.

I have prepared this book for you to give you the opportunity to discover exceptional recipes, keeping you healthy and adding with taste a rich source of protein.

But let's not waste any more time and start cooking our favorite meat right away.

BEEF, PORK AND LAMB RECIPES

BEEF SHAMI KABOB

Ingredients:

- 1 pound (454 g) beef chunks, chopped

- 1 teaspoon ginger paste

- ½ teaspoon ground cumin

- 2 cups water

- ¼ cup almond flour

- 1 egg, beaten

- 1 tablespoon coconut oil

Instructions

1. Put the beef chunks, ginger paste, ground cumin, and water in the Instant Pot.

2. Select Manual mode and set cooking time for 30 minutes on High Pressure.

3. When timer beeps, make a quick pressure release. Open the lid.

4. Drain the water from the meat. Transfer the beef in the blender. Add the almond flour and beaten egg. Blend until smooth. Shape the mixture into small meatballs.

5. Heat the coconut oil on Sauté mode and put the meatballs inside.

6. Cook for 2 minutes on each side or until golden brown.

7. Serve immediately.

Preparation Time: 15 minutes **Servings:** 4

Cooking Time: 35 minutes

Nutrition: calories: 179 fat: 9.5g protein: 20.1g carbs: 2.9g net carbs: 2.6g fiber: 0.3g

BEEF SHAWARMA AND VEGGIE SALAD BOWLS

Ingredients:

- 2 teaspoons olive oil

- 1½ pounds (680 g) beef flank steak, thinly sliced

- Sea salt and freshly ground black pepper, to taste

- 1 teaspoon cayenne pepper

- ½ teaspoon ground bay leaf

- ½ teaspoon ground allspice

- ½ teaspoon cumin, divided

- ½ cup Greek yogurt

- 2 tablespoons sesame oil

- 1 tablespoon fresh lime juice

- 2 English cucumbers, chopped

- 1 cup cherry tomatoes, halved

- 1 red onion, thinly sliced

- ½ head romaine lettuce, chopped

Instructions

1. Press the Sauté button to heat up the Instant Pot. Then, heat the olive oil and cook the beef for about 4 minutes.

2. Add all seasonings, 1½ cups of water, and secure the lid.

3. Choose Manual mode. Set the cook time for 15 minutes on High Pressure.

4. Once cooking is complete, use a natural pressure release. Carefully remove the lid.

5. Allow the beef to cool completely.

6. To make the dressing, whisk Greek yogurt, sesame oil, and lime juice in a mixing bowl.

7. Then, divide cucumbers, tomatoes, red onion, and romaine lettuce among four serving bowls. Dress the salad and top with the reserved beef flank steak. Serve warm.

Preparation Time: 10 minutes **Servings:** 4

Cooking Time: 19 minutes

Nutrition: calories: 367 fat: 19.1g protein: 39.5g carbs: 8.4g net carbs: 5.0g fiber: 3.4g

BEEF SHOULDER ROAST

Ingredients:

- 2 tablespoons peanut oil

- 2 pounds (907 g) shoulder roast

- ¼ cup coconut aminos

- 1 teaspoon porcini powder

- 1 teaspoon garlic powder

- 1 cup beef broth

- 2 cloves garlic, minced

- 2 tablespoons champagne vinegar

- ½ teaspoon hot sauce

- 1 teaspoon celery seeds

- 1 cup purple onions, cut into wedges

- 1 tablespoon flaxseed meal, plus 2 tablespoons water

Instructions

- Press the Sauté button to heat up the Instant Pot. Then, heat the peanut oil and cook the beef shoulder roast for 3 minutes on each side.

- In a mixing dish, combine coconut aminos, porcini powder, garlic powder, broth, garlic, vinegar, hot sauce, and celery seeds.

- Pour the broth mixture into the Instant Pot. Add the onions to the top.

- Secure the lid. Choose Meat/Stew mode and set cooking time for 40 minutes on High Pressure.

- Once cooking is complete, use a natural pressure release for 15 mintues, then release any remaining pressure. Carefully remove the lid.

- Make the slurry by mixing flaxseed meal with 2 tablespoons of water. Add the slurry to the Instant Pot.

- Press the Sauté button and allow it to cook until the cooking liquid is reduced and thickened slightly. Serve warm.

Preparation Time: 15 minutes **Servings:** 6

Cooking Time: 46 minutes

Nutrition: calories: 313 fat: 16.1g protein: 33.5g carbs: 6.5g net carbs: 3.1g fiber: 3.4g

BEEF STUFFED KALE ROLLS

Ingredients:

- 8 ounces (227 g) ground beef

- 1 teaspoon chives

- ¼ teaspoon cayenne pepper

- 4 kale leaves

- 1 tablespoon cream cheese

- ¼ cup heavy cream

- ½ cup chicken broth

Instructions

1. In the mixing bowl, combine the ground beef, chives, and cayenne pepper.

2. Then fill and roll the kale leaves with ground beef mixture.

3. Place the kale rolls in the Instant Pot.

4. Add cream cheese, heavy cream, and chicken broth. Close the lid.

5. Select Manual mode and set cooking time for 30 minutes on High Pressure

6. When timer beeps, make a quick pressure release. Open the lid.

7. Serve warm.

Preparation Time: 15 minutes **Servings:** 4

Cooking Time: 30 minutes

Nutrition: calories: 153 fat: 7.4g protein: 18.7g carbs: 2.2g net carbs: 1.9g fiber: 0.3g

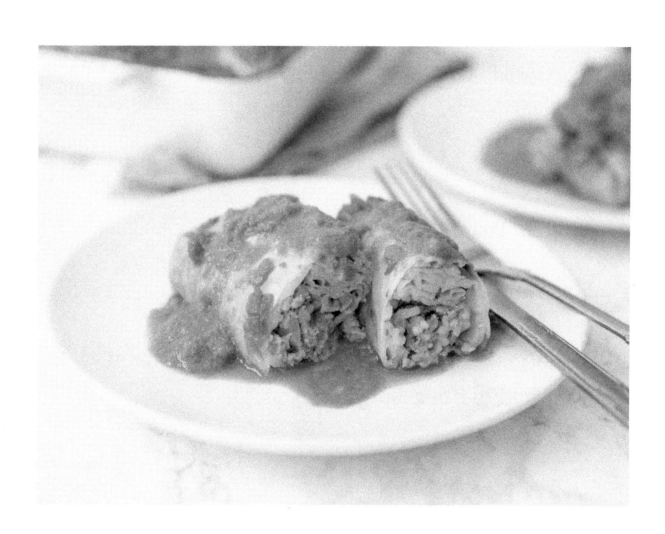

BEEF, BACON AND CAULIFLOWER RICE CASSEROLE

Ingredients:

- 2 cups fresh cauliflower florets

- 1 pound (454 g) ground beef

- 5 slices uncooked bacon, chopped

- 8 ounces (227 g) unsweetened tomato puree

- 1 cup shredded Cheddar cheese, divided

- 1 teaspoon garlic powder

- ½ teaspoon paprika

- ½ teaspoon sea salt

- ¼ teaspoon ground black pepper

- ¼ teaspoon celery seed

- 1 cup water

- 1 medium Roma tomato, sliced

Instructions

1. Spray a round soufflé dish with coconut oil cooking spray. Set aside.

2. Add the cauliflower florets to a food processor and pulse until a riced. Set aside.

3. Select Sauté mode. Once the pot is hot, crumble the ground beef into the pot and add the bacon. Sauté for 6 minutes or until the ground beef is browned and the bacon is cooked through.

4. Transfer the beef, bacon, and rendered fat to a large bowl.

5. Add the cauliflower rice, tomato puree ½ cup Cheddar cheese, garlic powder, paprika, sea salt, black pepper, and celery seed to the bowl with the beef and bacon. Mix well to combine.

6. Add the mixture to the prepared dish and use a spoon to press and smooth the mixture into an even layer.

7. Place the trivet in the Instant Pot and add the water to the bottom of the pot. Place the dish on top of the trivet.

8. Lock the lid. Set to Manual mode and adjust cooking time for twenty minutes on High Pressure.

9. When cooking is complete, quick release the pressure.

10. Open the lid. Arrange the tomato slices in a single layer on top of the casserole and sprinkle the remaining cheese over top.

11. Secure the lid and let the residual heat melt the cheese for 5 minutes.

12. Open the lid, remove the dish from the pot.

13. Transfer the casserole to a serving plate and slice into 5 equal-sized wedges. Serve warm.

Preparation Time: 15 minutes **Servings:** 5

Cooking Time: 26 minutes

Nutrition: calories: 350 fat: 22.7g protein: 30.0g carbs: 8.0g net carbs: 6.0g fiber: 2.0g

CILANTRO GARLIC PORK CHOPS

Ingredients:

- 1 pound boneless center-cut pork chops, pounded to ¼ inch thick

- Sea salt, for seasoning

- Freshly ground black pepper, for seasoning

- ¼ cup good-quality olive oil, divided

- ¼ cup finely chopped fresh cilantro

- 1 tablespoon minced garlic

- Juice of 1 lime

Instructions

1. Marinate the pork. Pat the pork chops dry and season them lightly with salt and pepper. Place them in a large bowl, add 2 tablespoons of the olive oil, and the cilantro, garlic, and lime juice. Toss to coat the chops. Cover the bowl and marinate the chops at room temperature for 30 minutes. Cook the pork. In a large skillet over medium-high heat, warm the remaining 2 tablespoons of olive oil. Add the pork chops in a single layer and fry them, turning them once, until they're just cooked through and still juicy, 6 to 7 minutes per side.

2. Serve. Divide the chops between four plates and serve them immediately.

Preparation Time: 10 Minutes **Servings:** 4

Cooking Time: 15 Minutes

Nutrition: Calories: 249 Total fat: 16g Total carbs: 2g Fiber: 0g; Net carbs: 2g Sodium: 261mg Protein: 25g

SPINACH FETA STUFFED PORK

Ingredients:

- 4 ounces crumbled feta cheese

- ¾ cup chopped frozen spinach, thawed and liquid squeezed out

- 3 tablespoons chopped Kalamata olives

- 4 (4-ounce) center pork chops, 2 inches thick

- Sea salt, for seasoning

- Freshly ground black pepper, for seasoning

- 3 tablespoons good-quality olive oil

Instructions

1. Preheat the oven. Set the oven temperature to 400°F.

2. Make the filling. In a small bowl, mix together the feta, spinach, and olives until everything is well combined.

3. Stuff the pork chops. Make a horizontal slit in the side of each chop to create a pocket, making sure you don't cut all the way

through. Stuff the filling equally between the chops and secure the slits with toothpicks. Lightly season the stuffed chops with salt and pepper.

4. Brown the chops. In a large oven-safe skillet over medium-high heat, warm the olive oil.

5. Add the chops and sear them until they're browned all over, about 10 minutes in total.

6. Roast the chops. Place the skillet in the oven and roast the chops for 20 minutes or until they're cooked through.

7. Serve. Let the meat rest for 10 minutes and then remove the toothpicks. Divide the pork chops between four plates and serve them immediately.

Preparation Time: 15 Minutes **Servings:** 4

Cooking Time: 30 Minutes

Nutrition: Calories: 342 Total fat: 24g Total carbs: 3g Fiber: 1g; Net carbs: 2g Sodium: 572mg Protein: 28g

COCONUT MILK GINGER MARINATED PORK TENDERLOIN

Ingredients:

- ¼ cup coconut oil, divided

- 1½ pounds boneless pork chops, about ¾ inch thick

- 1 tablespoon grated fresh ginger

- 2 teaspoons minced garlic

- 1 cup coconut milk

- 1 teaspoon chopped fresh basil

- Juice of 1 lime

- ½ cup shredded unsweetened coconut

Instructions

1. Brown the pork. In a large skillet over medium heat, warm 2 tablespoons of the coconut oil. Add the pork chops to the skillet and brown them all over, turning them several times, about 10 minutes in total.

2. Braise the pork. Move the pork to the side of the skillet and add the remaining 2 tablespoons of coconut oil. Add the ginger and garlic and sauté until they've softened, about 2 minutes. Stir in the coconut milk, basil, and lime juice and move the pork back to the center of the skillet. Cover the skillet and simmer until the pork is just cooked through and very tender, 12 to 15 minutes.

3. Serve. Divide the pork chops between four plates and top them with the shredded coconut.

Preparation Time: 5 Minutes **Servings:** 4

Cooking Time: 25 Minutes

Nutrition: Calories: 479 Total fat: 38g Total carbs: 6g Fiber: 3g; Net carbs: 3g Sodium: 318mg Protein: 32g

GRILLED PORK CHOPS WITH GREEK SALSA

Ingredients:

- ¼ cup good-quality olive oil, divided

- 1 tablespoon red wine vinegar

- 3 teaspoons chopped fresh oregano, divided

- 1 teaspoon minced garlic

- 4 (4-ounce) boneless center-cut loin pork chops

- ½ cup halved cherry tomatoes

- ½ yellow bell pepper, diced

- ½ English cucumber, chopped

- ¼ red onion, chopped

- 1 tablespoon balsamic vinegar

- Sea salt, for seasoning

- Freshly ground black pepper, for seasoning

Instructions

1. Marinate the pork. In a medium bowl, stir together 3 tablespoons of the olive oil, the vinegar, 2 teaspoons of the oregano, and the garlic. Add the pork chops to the bowl, turning them to get them coated with the marinade. Cover the bowl and place it in the refrigerator for 30 minutes.

2. Make the salsa. While the pork is marinating, in a medium bowl, stir together the remaining 1 tablespoon of olive oil, the tomatoes, yellow bell pepper, cucumber, red onion, vinegar, and the remaining 1 teaspoon of oregano. Season the salsa with salt and pepper. Set the bowl aside.

3. Grill the pork chops. Heat a grill to medium-high heat. Remove the pork chops from the marinade and grill them until just cooked through, 6 to 8 minutes per side.

4. Serve. Rest the pork for 5 minutes. Divide the pork between four plates and serve them with a generous scoop of the salsa.

Preparation Time: 15 Minutes **Servings:** 4

Cooking Time: 15 Minutes

Nutrition: Calories: 277 Total fat: 19g Total carbs: 4g Fiber: 1g; Net carbs: 3g Sodium: 257mg; Protein: 25g

GRILLED HERBED PORK KEBABS

Ingredients:

- ¼ cup good-quality olive oil

- 1 tablespoon minced garlic

- 2 teaspoons dried oregano

- 1 teaspoon dried basil

- 1 teaspoon dried parsley

- ½ teaspoon sea salt

- 1/4 teaspoon freshly ground black pepper

- 1 (1-pound) pork tenderloin, cut into 1½-inch pieces

Instructions

1. Marinate the pork. In a medium bowl, stir together the olive oil, garlic, oregano, basil, parsley, salt, and pepper. Add the pork pieces and toss to coat them in the marinade. Cover the bowl and place it in the refrigerator for 2 to 4 hours.

2. Make the kebabs. Divide the pork pieces between four skewers, making sure to not crowd the meat.

3. Grill the kebabs. Preheat your grill to medium-high heat. Grill the skewers for about 12 minutes, turning to cook all sides of the pork, until the pork is cooked through.

4. Serve. Rest the skewers for 5 minutes. Divide the skewers between four plates and serve them immediately.

Preparation Time: 10 Minutes **Servings:** 4

Cooking Time: 15 Minutes

Nutrition: Calories: 261 Total fat: 18g Total carbs: 1g Fiber: 0g; Net carbs: 1g Sodium: 60mg Protein: 24

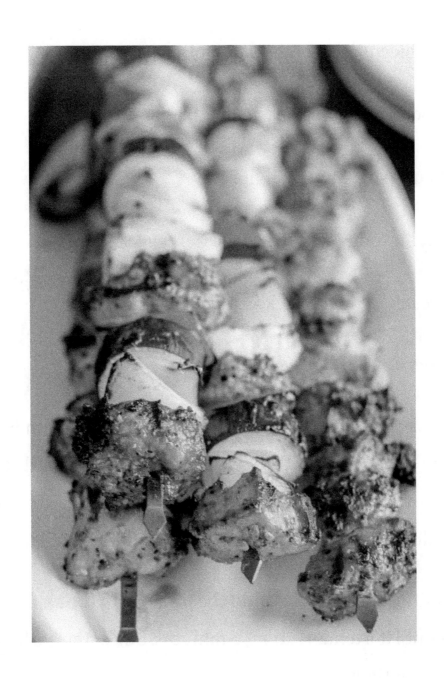

ITALIAN SAUSAGE BROCCOLI SAUTÉ

Ingredients:

- 2 tablespoons good-quality olive oil

- 1 pound Italian sausage meat, hot or mild

- 4 cups small broccoli florets

- 1 tablespoon minced garlic

- Freshly ground black pepper, for seasoning

Instructions

1. Cook the sausage. In a large skillet over medium heat, warm the olive oil. Add the sausage and sauté it until it's cooked through, 8 to 10 minutes. Transfer the sausage to a plate with a slotted spoon and set the plate aside.

2. Sauté the vegetables. Add the broccoli to the skillet and sauté it until it's tender, about 6 minutes. Stir in the garlic and sauté for another 3 minutes.

3. Finish the dish. Return the sausage to the skillet and toss to combine it with the other ingredients. Season the mixture with pepper.

4. Serve. Divide the mixture between four plates and serve it immediately.

Preparation Time: 10 Minutes **Servings:** 4

Cooking Time: 20 Minutes

Nutrition: Calories: 486 Total fat: 43g Total carbs: 7g Fiber: 2g; Net carbs: 5g Sodium: 513mg Protein: 19g

CLASSIC SAUSAGE AND PEPPERS

Ingredients:

- 1½ pounds sweet Italian sausages (or hot if you prefer)

- 2 tablespoons good-quality olive oil

- 1 red bell pepper, cut into thin strips

- 1 yellow bell pepper, cut into thin strips

- 1 orange bell pepper, cut into thin strips

- 1 red onion, thinly sliced

- 1 tablespoon minced garlic

- ½ cup white wine

- Sea salt, for seasoning

- Freshly ground black pepper, for seasoning

Instructions

1. Cook the sausage. Preheat a grill to medium-high and grill the sausages, turning them several times, until they're cooked through, about 12 minutes in total. Let the sausages rest for 15 minutes and then cut them into 2-inch pieces.

2. Sauté the vegetables. In a large skillet over medium-high heat, warm the olive oil. Add the red, yellow, and orange bell peppers, and the red onion and garlic and sauté until they're tender, about 10 minutes.

3. Finish the dish. Add the sausage to the skillet along with the white wine and sauté for 10 minutes.

4. Serve. Divide the mixture between four plates, season it with salt and pepper, and serve.

Preparation Time: 10 Minutes **Servings:** 6

Cooking Time: 35 Minutes

Nutrition: Calories: 450 Total fat: 40g Total carbs: 5g Fiber: 1g; Net carbs: 4g Sodium: 554mg Protein: 17g

LEMON-INFUSED PORK RIB ROAST

Ingredients:

- ¼ cup good-quality olive oil

- Zest and juice of 1 lemon

- Zest and juice of 1 orange

- 4 rosemary sprigs, lightly crushed

- 4 thyme sprigs, lightly crushed

- 1 (4-bone) pork rib roast, about 2½ pounds

- 6 garlic cloves, peeled

- Sea salt, for seasoning

- Freshly ground black pepper, for seasoning

Instructions

1. Make the marinade. In a large bowl, combine the olive oil, lemon zest, lemon juice, orange zest, orange juice, rosemary sprigs, and thyme sprigs.

2. Marinate the roast. Use a small knife to make six 1-inch-deep slits in the fatty side of the roast. Stuff the garlic cloves in the slits. Put the roast in the bowl with the marinade and turn it to coat it well with the marinade. Cover the bowl and refrigerate it overnight, turning the roast in the marinade several times.

3. Preheat the oven. Set the oven temperature to 350°F.

4. Roast the pork. Remove the pork from the marinade and season it with salt and pepper, then put it in a baking dish and let it come to room temperature. Roast the pork until it's cooked through (145°F to 160°F internal temperature), about 1 hour. Throw out any leftover marinade.

5. Serve. Let the pork rest for 10 minutes, then cut it into slices and arrange the slices on a platter. Serve it warm.

Preparation Time: 10 Minutes **Servings:** 6

Cooking Time: 1 Hour

Nutrition: Calories: 403 Total fat: 30g Total carbs: 1g Fiber: 0g; Net carbs: 1g Sodium: 113mg Protein: 30g

PORK MEATBALL PARMESAN

Ingredients:

For The Meatballs:

- 1¼ Pounds ground pork

- ½ cup almond flour

- ½ cup Parmesan cheese

- 1 egg, lightly beaten

- 1 tablespoon chopped fresh parsley

- 1 teaspoon minced garlic

- 1 teaspoon chopped fresh oregano

- ¼ teaspoon sea salt

- 1/8 teaspoon freshly ground black pepper

- 2 tablespoons good-quality olive oil

FOR THE PARMIGIANA:

- 1 cup sugar-free tomato sauce

- 1 cup shredded mozzarella cheese

Instructions

1. Make the meatballs. In a large bowl, mix together the ground pork, almond flour, Parmesan, egg, parsley, garlic, oregano, salt, and pepper until everything is well mixed. Roll the pork mixture into 1½-inch meatballs.

2. Cook the meatballs. In a large skillet over medium-high heat, warm the olive oil. Add the meatballs to the skillet and cook them, turning them several times, until they're completely cooked through, about 15 minutes in total.

TO MAKE THE PARMIGIANA:

1. Preheat the oven. Set the oven temperature to 350°F.

2. Assemble the parmigiana. Transfer the meatballs to a 9-by-9-inch baking dish and top them with the tomato sauce. Sprinkle with the mozzarella and bake for 15 minutes or until the cheese is melted and golden.

3. Serve. Divide the meatballs and sauce between six bowls and serve it immediately.

Preparation Time: 15 Minutes **Servings:** 6

Cooking Time: 30 Minutes

Nutrition: Calories: 403 Total fat: 32g Total carbs: 1g Fiber: 0g; Net carbs: 1g Sodium: 351mg Protein: 25g

CHIPOTLE LAMB RIBS

Ingredients:

- 2-pound lamb ribs

- 1 tablespoon chipotle pepper, minced

- 2 tablespoons sesame oil

- 1 teaspoon apple cider vinegar

Instructions

1. Mix lamb ribs with all ingredients and leave to marinate for 10 minutes.

2. Then transfer the lamb ribs and all marinade in the baking tray and cook the meat in the oven at 360F for 40 minutes. Flip the ribs on another side after 20 minutes of cooking.

Preparation Time: 15 minutes **Servings:** 6

Cooking Time: 20 minutes

Nutrition: Calories 392 Fat 24.7 Fiber 0 Carbs 0.2 Protein 39.6

LAMB AND PECAN SALAD

Ingredients:

- 2 lamb chops

- 1 tablespoon sesame oil

- 2 pecans, chopped

- 2 cups lettuce, chopped

- 1 teaspoon cayenne pepper

- 1 tablespoon avocado oil

Instructions

1. Sprinkle the lamb chops with cayenne pepper and put in the hot skillet.

2. Add sesame oil and roast the meat for 4 minutes per side.

3. Then chops the lamb chops and put them in the salad bowl.

4. Add all remaining ingredients and carefully mix the salad.

Preparation Time: 10 minutes **Servings:** 4

Cooking Time: 10 minutes

Nutrition: Calories 168 Fat 12.1 Fiber 1 Carbs 2.3 Protein 12.9

HOT SAUCE LAMB

Ingredients:

- 2 teaspoons paprika

- 1-pound lamb fillet, chopped

- 1 tablespoon coconut oil

- 4 tablespoons keto hot sauce

- ½ cup of water

Instructions

1. Pour water in the saucepan and bring it to boil.

2. Add lamb and boil it for 20 minutes.

3. After this, preheat the skillet well.

4. Add boiled lamb fillet, coconut oil, and paprika.

5. Roast the ingredients for 6 minutes per side or until the meat is light brown.

6. Then add hot sauce and carefully mix the meal.

Preparation Time: 10 minutes **Servings:** 4

Cooking Time: 35 minutes

Nutrition: Calories 245 Fat 11.9 Fiber 0.4 Carbs 0.8 Protein 32.1

MUSTARD LAMB CHOPS

Ingredients:

- 1 cup spinach

- 3 tablespoons mustard

- 2 tablespoons sesame oil

- ½ teaspoon ground turmeric

- 4 lamb chops

Instructions

1. Blend the spinach and mix it with mustard, sesame oil, and ground turmeric.

2. Then rub the lamb chops with the mustard mixture and put in the baking pan.

3. Bake the meat at 355F for 40 minutes. Flip the meat after 20 minutes of cooking.

Preparation Time: 10 minutes **Servings:** 4

Cooking Time: 40 minutes

Nutrition: Calories 102 Fat 9.3 Fiber 1.5 Carbs 3.4 Protein 2.3

GINGER LAMB CHOPS

Ingredients:

- 6 lamb chops

- 1 tablespoon keto tomato paste

- 1 teaspoon minced ginger

- 2 tablespoons avocado oil

- 1 teaspoon plain yogurt

Instructions

1. Mix plain yogurt with keto tomato paste and minced ginger.

2. Then put the lamb chops in the yogurt mixture and marinate for 10-15 minutes.

3. After this, transfer the mixture in the tray, add avocado oil, and cook the meat at 360F in the oven for 30 minutes.

Preparation Time: 15 minutes **Servings:** 6

Cooking Time: 30 minutes

Nutrition: Calories 330 Fat 26.6 Fiber 0.4 Carbs 1 Protein 19.3

PARMESAN LAMB

Ingredients:

- 4 lamb chops

- 2 oz. Parmesan, grated

- ½ cup plain yogurt

- 3 scallions, sliced

- 1 tablespoon butter, softened

Instructions

1. Melt the butter in the saucepan. Add scallions and roast it for 3-4 minutes.

2. Then stir the scallions and add lamb chops.

3. Roast them for 2 minutes per side.

4. Add yogurt and close the lid. Cook the meat for 10 minutes.

5. After this, top the meat with Parmesan and cook it for 2 minutes more.

Preparation Time: 10 minutes **Servings:** 4

Cooking Time: 20 minutes

Nutrition: Calories 262 Fat 12.6 Fiber 0.6 Carbs 5.2 Protein 30.5

CLOVE LAMB

Ingredients:

- 1 teaspoon ground clove

- 2 tablespoons butter

- 1 teaspoon ground paprika

- 1 teaspoon dried rosemary

- ¼ cup of water

- 12 oz. lamb fillet

Instructions

1. In the shallow bowl, mix ground clove with ground paprika, and dried rosemary.

2. Rub the lamb fillet with spices and grease with butter.

3. Then put the meat in the hot skillet and roast it for 5 minutes per side on the low heat.

4. Add water. Close the lid and cook the lamb on medium heat for 15 minutes.

Preparation Time: 10 minutes **Servings:** 4

Cooking Time: 25 minutes

Nutrition: Calories 55 Fat 6 Fiber 0.5 Carbs 0.8 Protein 0.2

CARROT LAMB ROAST

Ingredients:

- 1-pound lamb loin

- 1 carrot, chopped

- 1 teaspoon dried thyme

- 2 tablespoons coconut oil

- 1 teaspoon salt

Instructions

1. Put all ingredients in the baking tray, mix well.

2. Bake the mixture in the preheated to 360F oven for 40 minutes.

Preparation Time: 10 minutes **Servings:** 4

Cooking Time: 40 minutes

Nutrition: Calories 295 Fat 17.9 Fiber 0.5 Carbs 1.7 Protein 30.3

LAMB AND CELERY CASSEROLE

Ingredients:

- ¼ cup celery stalk, chopped

- 2 lamb chops, chopped

- ½ cup Mozzarella, shredded

- 1 teaspoon butter

- ¼ cup coconut cream

- 1 teaspoon taco seasonings

Instructions

1. Mix lamb chops with taco seasonings and put in the casserole mold.

2. Add celery stalk, coconut cream, and shredded mozzarella.

3. Then add butter and cook the casserole in the preheated to 360F oven for 45 minutes.

Preparation Time: 10 minutes **Servings:** 2

Cooking Time: 45 minutes

Nutrition: Calories 283 Fat 19.3 Fiber 0.9 Carbs 3.3 Protein 24.8

LAMB IN ALMOND SAUCE

Preparation Time: 10 minutes **Servings:** 6

Cooking Time: 30 minutes

Ingredients:

- 14 oz. lamb fillet, cubed

- 1 cup organic almond milk

- 1 teaspoon almond flour

- 1 teaspoon ground nutmeg

- ½ teaspoon ground cardamom

- 1 tablespoon olive oil

- 1 tablespoon lemon juice

- 1 tablespoon butter

- ½ teaspoon minced garlic

Instructions

- Preheat the olive oil in the saucepan.

- Meanwhile, mix lamb, ground nutmeg, ground cardamom, and minced garlic.

- Put the lamb in the hot olive oil. Roast the meat for 2 minutes per side.

- Then add butter, lemon juice, and almond milk. Carefully mix the mixture.

- Cook the meal for 15 minutes on medium heat.

- Then add almond flour, stir well and simmer the meal for 10 minutes more.

Nutrition: Calories 258 Fat 19 Fiber 1.1 Carbs 2.7 Protein 19.7

Sweet Leg of Lamb

Ingredients:

- 2 pounds lamb leg

- 1 tablespoon Erythritol

- 3 tablespoons coconut milk

- 1 teaspoon chili flakes

- 1 teaspoon ground turmeric

- 1 teaspoon cayenne pepper

- 3 tablespoons coconut oil

Instructions

1. In the shallow bowl, mix cayenne pepper, ground turmeric, chili flakes, and Erythritol.

2. Rub the lamb leg with spices.

3. Melt the coconut oil in the saucepan.

4. Add lamb leg and roast it for 10 minutes per side on low heat.

5. After this, add coconut milk and cook the meal for 30 minutes on low heat. Flip the meat on another side from time to time.

Preparation Time: 10 minutes **Servings:** 6

Cooking Time: 45 minutes

Nutrition: Calories 350 Fat 18.8 Fiber 0.3 Carbs 0.8 Protein 42.8

COCONUT LAMB SHOULDER

Ingredients:

- 2-pound lamb shoulder

- 1 teaspoon ground cumin

- 2 tablespoons butter

- ¼ cup of coconut milk

- 1 teaspoon coconut shred

- ½ cup kale, chopped

Instructions

1. Put all ingredients in the saucepan and mix well.

2. Close the lid and cook the meal on low heat for 75 minutes.

Preparation Time: 10 minutes **Servings:** 5

Cooking Time: 75 minutes

Nutrition: Calories 414 Fat 21.2 Fiber 0.5 Carbs 1.7 Protein 51.5

LAVENDER LAMB

Ingredients:

- 4 lamb chops

- 1 teaspoon dried lavender

- 2 tablespoons butter

- 1 teaspoon cumin seeds

- 1 cup of water

Instructions

1. Toss the butter in the saucepan and melt it.

2. Add lamb chops and roast them for 3 minutes.

3. Then add dried lavender, cumin seeds, and water.

4. Close the lid and cook the meat for 30 minutes on medium-low heat.

Preparation Time: 10 minutes **Servings:** 4

Cooking Time: 35 minutes

Nutrition: Calories 211 Fat 12.1 Fiber 0.1 Carbs 0.2 Protein 24

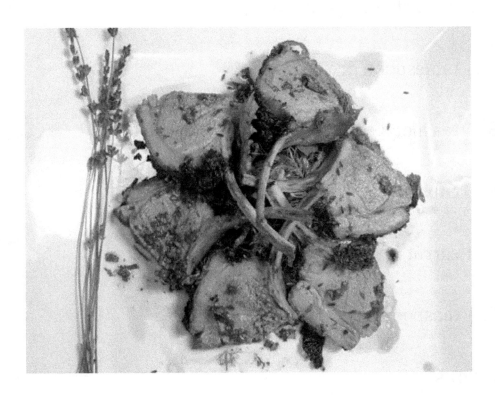

DILL LAMB SHANK

Ingredients:

1. 3 lamb shanks (4 oz. each)

2. 1 tablespoon dried dill

3. 1 teaspoon peppercorns

4. 3 cups of water

5. 1 carrot, chopped

6. 1 teaspoon salt

Instructions

1. Bring the water to boil.

2. Add lamb shank, dried dill, peppercorns, carrot, and salt.

3. Close the lid and cook the meat in medium heat for 40 minutes.

Preparation Time: 10 minutes **Servings:** 3

Cooking Time: 40 minutes

Nutrition: Calories 224 Fat 84 Fiber 0.8 Carbs 3 Protein 32.3

MEXICAN LAMB CHOPS

Ingredients:

- 4 lamb chops

- 1 tablespoon Mexican seasonings

- 2 tablespoons sesame oil

- 1 teaspoon butter

Instructions

1. Rub the lamb chops with Mexican seasonings.

2. Then melt the butter in the skillet. Add sesame oil.

3. Then add lamb chops and roast them for 7 minutes per side on medium heat.

Preparation Time: 10 minutes **Servings:** 4

Cooking Time: 15 minutes

Nutrition: Calories 323 Fat 14 Fiber 0 Carbs 1.1 Protein 24.1

VEGAN RECIPES

PESTO SPAGHETTI WITH ZUCCHINI (ZOODLES)

Ingredients

8. 2 medium-sized zucchini, spiral-shaped (see notes below)

9. ⅓ cup vegan pesto, + more if necessary

10. ½ red onion, finely sliced and cut in half

11. 6 mushrooms, thinly sliced (cremini or white bud)

12. 10 cherry tomatoes, cut in half

13. 2 garlic cloves, finely chopped

14. 2 tsp olive oil

15. salt to taste

16. freshly ground black pepper (optional)

17. chopped red pepper (optional)

18. cashew cream (optional drizzle)

Instructions

1. In a skillet, heat the olive oil over medium to high heat.

2. Add chopped garlic, chopped onions, and chopped mushrooms. Add about ¼ tsp salt.

3. Bake until vegetables are tender and soft, but crisp. Keep in mind that the water is cooked when the mushrooms are cooked. Put aside.

4. Quickly clean the pan with a damp towel.

5. Heat ¼ cup pesto, add the zucchini spaghetti in a spiral shape, and cook for 1 to 2 min over medium heat to cook quickly.

6. Add fried onions/mushrooms and halves of cherry tomatoes.

7. Add the rest of the pesto. If necessary, you can add more pesto than the amount indicated above. (optional) Add a dash of cream if using it.

8. Cook another 1 to 2 min, stirring regularly.

9. Season with salt freshly ground black pepper and crushed red pepper (if used).

Prep time: 10 min; **Servings:** 3

Macros: Cal 226n Cal from Fat 176 Fat 19.6g Saturated Fat 1.9g Carbs 11.4g Fiber 3.1g Sugar 6.3g Protein 4.5g

INSTANT POT CAULIFLOWER MUSHROOM RISOTTO

Ingredients

- 1 cup medium-sized gold cauliflower 4-5 cups pre-cooked fresh gold frozen cauliflower

- 1 Tbsp coconut oil for AIP or sensitivity to dairy products, 1 small onion, diced, 1 lb of small shiitake mushrooms, sliced or cremini or white mushrooms

- 3 cloves oFinely chopped garlic, 2 Tbsp coconut amino acids, 1 full cup coconut milk

- 1 cup bone broth or chicken broth or vegetable broth, ¼ cup nutritional yeast

- ½ tsp or more sea salt, to taste, 2 Tbsp tapioca starch

- Ground black pepper to taste (skip for AIP)

- Chopped parsley to decorate

Instructions

1. Remove cauliflower leaves and cut the flowers from the roots.

2. Use a cheese grater or food processor with a grater and grated cauliflower to the size of the rice.

3. Add the butter or coconut oil to the prepared pan and set it to "Sautéed." Let's cool for 5 min and cover the bottom of the pan.

4. Add the onion, mushrooms and garlic and cook, stirring, for 7 min, until the mushrooms are sweaty and soft.

5. Add the coconut amino acids and sauté for 5 min until the vegetables are brown. Turn off the instant pot.

6. Add the cauliflower rice and coconut milk. bone broth, nutritional yeast, and sea salt. Stir together.

7. Close the lid, make sure the valve is closed and set the instant pot to "Manual" for 2 min

8. Release the pressure valve and open the lid.

9. Sprinkle tapioca starch on the risotto and stir until thickened. Add more salt if you wish. Add ground black pepper if you are using it.

10. Serve hot, sprinkled with parsley chopped.

Prep time: 15 min; **Servings:** 4

Macros: Cal 299.05 Cal from Fat 172 Fat 19.15g Saturated Fat 15.12g Cholesterol 9.6mg Sodium 546.4mg Carbs 27.61g Fiber 8.31g Sugar 8.64g Protein 10.62g

CAULIFLOWER STEAKS

Ingredients

- 1 big cauliflower

- 3 Tbsp split olive oil

- ¼ cup parsley chopped

- ¼ cup chopped raw pumpkin seeds

- Pink Himalayan salt to taste

- black pepper to taste

Instructions

1. Preheat the oven to 400° C and line a baking sheet with parchment paper.

2. Cut the cauliflower stalk to rest on a flat surface. The number oFillets depends on the size and condition of the cauliflower.

3. Place the cauliflower on the baking sheet coated and sprinkle with 2 Tbsp olive oil. Sprinkle the salt with a pinch of salt and pepper. Bake 30 min or until cauliflower is golden.

4. While cooking cauliflower, mix remaining Tbsp of olive with parsley and pumpkin seeds and season with salt and pepper. When the cauliflower is ready to fry, for the right amount of tahini lemon vinaigrette and cover it with the spice mixture.

Prep time:5 min; **Servings:** 2-4

Macros: Cal 350 Carbs 50 g Fat 7 g Protein 22 g

EVERYDAY LEMON TAHINI

Ingredients

- ¼ cup + 1 Tbsp lukewarm filtered water

- ¼ cup tahini

- 1 garlic clove, diced

- 2 Tbsp lemon juice

- ½ tsp maple syrup {see comments}

- ¼ tsp pink Himalayan salt

- A pinch of of black pepper

Instructions

1. Mix all ingredients in a blender

2. Blender until smooth.

Prep time:5 min; **Servings:** 6

Macros: Cal 140 Carbs 4g Fat 11g Protein 8g

KALE TOFU STIR FRY

Ingredients

- 1 block of extra healthy cubic tofu

- 6 cups chopped kale

- 1 clove garlic minced

- 2 Tbsp liquid amino acids of Bragg or soy sauce

- 1 Tbsp sesame seeds

Instructions

1. Drain the tofu: wrap a block of tofu in a paper towel. Drain the tofu for about 15-20 min

2. Spray the pan with nonstick cooking spray. Add chopped garlic and bring to medium heat.

3. Add the tofu and form an even layer. Bake 2 min

4. Add kale and liquid amino acids and cook for 8 to 10 minutes, stirring occasionally.

5. Cover with sesame seeds and enjoy!

Prep time: 10 min; **Servings:** 3

Macros: Cal 232 Fat 12 g Saturated fat 2 g Sodium 1001 mg Carbs 7 g Fiber 6 g Protein 26 g

VEGAN KETO WALNUT CHILI

Ingredients

6. 2 Tbsp extra virgin olive oil

7. 5 thinly sliced celery stalks 2 garlic cloves, finely chopped 1 ½ tsp ground cinnamon

8. 2 tsp chili powder 4 tsp ground cumin

9. 1½ smoked pepper tsp 2 large pickled chipotle peppers

10. 2 finely chopped green peppers

11. 2 diced zucchini

12. 8 g of chopped mushrooms in a food processor 1 ½ Tbsp tomato puree 1 can of 15 oz tomato cubes 3 cups of water ½ cup coconut milk 2½ cups grated soy meat

13. 1 cup chopped raw walnuts

14. Tbsp unsweetened cocoa powder

15. Salt and pepper to taste

To serve:

3. 2 Tbsp fresh coriander leaves

4. 1 sliced avocado

5. 2 Tbsp sliced radish.

Instructions

1. Heat the oil in a large saucepan over medium heat. Add celery and cook for 4 min Add garlic, cinnamon, chili powder, cumin, and pepper and stir until fragrant, about 2 minutes more.

2. Add pepper, zucchini, mushrooms, and cook for 5 min

3. Add the chipotle, tomato puree, tomatoes, water, coconut milk, soy meat, nuts, and cocoa powder. Reduce heat to medium-low and simmer for about 20-25 min until thickened and vegetables are tender.

4. Season with salt and pepper. Cover with avocado, radish, and coriander.

Prep time:10 min; **Servings:** 4

Macros: Cal 353

AIR FRYER BUFFALO CAULIFLOWER WINGS

Ingredients

- 3-4 Tbsp hot sauce

- 1 Tbsp almond flour

- 1 Tbsp avocado oil

- Salt to taste

- 1 medium-sized cauliflower, washed and thoroughly dried

Instructions

1. Preheat the fryer to 400° F.

2. Mix hot sauce, almond flour, avocado oil, and salt in a large bowl.

3. Add the cauliflower and mix until covered.

4. Put half of the cauliflower in the fryer and cook for 12 to 15 min (or until it is crisp on the edges with a small cock or reaches the desired level).

5. Be sure to open the fryer and shake the fry basket halfway to rotate the cauliflower. Delete and book.

6. Add the second portion, but cook 2 to 3 min less.

Prep time:5 min; **Servings:** 4

Macros: Cal 48 | Carbs 1 g | Fat 4 g Sodium 265 mg | Potassium 94 mg Vitamin A: 15 IU | Vitamin C: 20.2 mg | Calcium: 10 mg Iron: 0.2 mg

GRAIN FREE GRANOLA

Ingredients

- 1 cup nuts and seeds

- 1 Tbsp agave syrup or sweetener of your choice

- ½ tsp vanilla extract

- 1 tsp almond extract

- 1 Tbsp melted coconut oil

- ¼ cup coconut chips

Instructions

1. Preheat the oven to 325° F.

2. Mix the agave syrup, extract vanilla, almond extract, and coconut oil in a bowl. Microwave 20-30 seconds to combine.

3. For the mixture over the nuts and seeds (no coconut chips) and mix well. Bake 10 min. Return and cook for 5 min Add the coconut chips and cook another 5 min.

Prep time: 10 min; **Servings:** 4

Macros: Cal 299 | Carbs 14 g Protein 6g Fat 25 g Saturated Fat 8 g Cholesterol 0 mg Sodium 6 mg Potassium 243 mg Fiber 4 g Sugar 4g Calcium: 25 mg Iron: 1.5 mg

KETO PEANUT BUTTER RAMEN

Ingredients

Sweet and spicy peanut sauce

- ¼ cup all-natural peanut butter (no added sugar, crisp or fresh)

- 1 tsp sambal oelek (add more if you like spicy)

- 1 ½ Tbsp soy sauce

- 1 tsp Truvia or another sugar-free sweetener that you like

Noodles and toppings

- 1 pack of House Foods Shirataki noodles

- 1 block of extra healthy tofu (about 100 g)

- 1 Tbsp coconut oil

- 1-2 chopped green onions

- 1 chopped cayenne pepper

- sesame seed drizzle (optional)

Instructions

1. Cut the tofu into large cubes and heat frying pan over medium heat. Add the coconut oil (1 Tbsp) and add it to the tofu. Stir so that the tofu does not stick. Once the tofu starts to turn a bit brown, turn it on with more soy sauce and stir. Remove the fire and reserve. You want the tofu to have a crispy exterior, but a sweet center.

2. Boil water (2 cups are enough). While the water boils, put the peanut butter (4 Tbsp) in a large bowl with the sambal oelek (chili paste), soy sauce (1 Tbsp) and the Truvia (1 tsp)).

3. Slowly add ⅓ cup boiled water into the large bowl. Mix well to emulsify. Depending on how you are, you may need a little more hot water or less. You are looking for a sauce that is neither thick nor liquid.

4. Remove the noodles from the package and place it in the microwave for 2 min Add the noodles to the peanut sauce and mix. When combined, sesame seeds, soy sauce, and chopped cayenne pepper.

Prep time: 10 min; **Servings:** 1

Macros: Cal 574 | Carbs 13.5 g | Protein 23 g | Fat 49 g | Saturated Fat 15.5 g Fiber 9 g

CURRY CABBAGE

Ingredients

- 1 lb of green cabbage, washed

- 2 Tbsp oil coconut or ¼ cup water/vegetable broth

- ½ cup chopped onion

- 2 garlic cloves, finely chopped

- 1 tsp ground coriander 1 tsp ground turmeric 1 tsp dried thyme leaves or 2 sprigs oFresh thyme

- ½ tsp cumin 1 chopped carrot

- 1-14 g of coconut milk ½ cup water 3/4 tsp sea salt, or to taste

Instructions

1. Cut cabbage into strips 1 inch thick, set aside in a bowl.

2. Heat the oil in a large saucepan over medium heat.

3. Add the onion and garlic and cook until tender, stirring for about 3 min

4. Add coriander, turmeric, thyme, caraway, carrot, cabbage, and stir. Add cocoon milk, water, and boil.

5. Cover the pan and simmer and cook for about 20 min or until the sauce thickens.

6. Delicious served with brown rice or baked potatoes and a salad!

Prep time: 10 min; **Servings:** 4

Macros: Macros: 171 / 715 kJ Fat 13 g Protein 3 g Carbohydrate: 12 g

VEGAN ZUCCHINI PASTA ALFREDO

Ingredients

- 2 medium-sized spiral zucchini

- 1-2 TB vegan parmesan (optional)

- Quick Alfredo sauce

- Soak ½ cup raw water for a few hours or 10 min in boiling water

- 2 Tbsp of lemon juice

- Nutritional yeast 3 TB

- 2 tsp white miso

- 1 tsp onion powder

- ½ tsp garlic powder

- ¼ to ½ cup water

Instructions

3. Zucchini noodles spiral.

4. Add all ingredients in a blender (starting with ¼ cup water) and mix until smooth. If your sauce is too thick, add 1 more Tbsp water.

5. Cover the zucchini noodles with Alfredo sauce and, if desired, a vegan parmesan.

Prep time: 5 min; **Servings:** 6

Macros: Cal 225 Cal from fat 144 Fat 16 g Carbs 19 g Fiber 6 g Protein 14 g

VEGAN QUICHE MUGS

Ingredients

- 1 extra stable tofu block (14 oz)

- 3 Tbsp water

- 1 Tbsp tomato sauce

- 2 Tbsp Dijon mustard

- 1 Tbsp lemon juice

- 1 Tbsp cornflour

- ½ cup nutritional yeast

- 2 tsp garlic herbs

Instructions

1. Preheat the oven to 350° F, cover the muffin pan with nonstick mussels or spray with nonstick cooking spray and set aside.

2. Mix all ingredients except green leafy vegetables in a blender and blend until smooth. Add more water if necessary, to facilitate mixing.

3. For the contents of the blender into a large mixing bowl, add green leafy vegetables and stir.

4. Spoon in the form of a muffin.

5. Bake for 30 to 35 min or until the edges begin to brown.

Prep time: 10 min; **Servings:** 12

Macros: Cal 57 Cal from fat 18 Fat 2 g Carbs 5 g Fiber 2 g Protein 6 g

CURRIED TOMATO SOUP

Ingredients

- 28 0z (800 g) chopped fresh tomatoes

- 1/5 cup (150 g) of cauliflower flowers

- 4 onions (chopped onions), finely chopped

- 1 Tbsp sweet curry powder

- 1 tsp ginger puree

- 1 tsp garlic puree

- 2 cups (500 mL) warm vegetable broth

- salt and pepper

Instructions

3. Add all the ingredients to the slow cooker and mix.

4. Cover and cook at high temperature for 3 hours.

5. Let the tomatoes cool for a while, then mash it in a blender, adjust the herbs, and serve.

Prep time:5 min; **Servings:** 4

Macros: Cal 54 | Carbs 12 g | Protein 2g | Sodium 758 mg Potassium 457 mg | Fiber 3g | Sugar 6g

LEMON TURMERIC ROASTED CAULIFLOWER

Ingredients

- 1 cup cauliflower

- 2 Tbsp chopped parsley

- Lemon and turmeric vinaigrette

- 3 Tbsp avocado oil

- 2 Tbsp lemon juice

- 3 cloves of garlic, finely chopped

- 1 tsp turmeric powder

- ½ tsp sea salt

Instructions

1. Preheat oven to 425 F.

2. Chop the cauliflower into bite-size bunches.

3. Beat the ingredients with the lemon-turmeric vinaigrette.

4. Place the cauliflower flowers in a large bowl and mix with the vinaigrette.

5. Spread cauliflower on a baking sheet in 1 layer.

6. Roast in the oven for 20-25 min

7. Sprinkle with chopped parsley before serving.

Prep time: 5 min; **Servings:** 4

Macros: Cal 107 Cal from Fat 90 Fat 10 g Saturated Fat 1 g Carbs 3 g

LEMON BRUSSELS SPROUTS WITH GARLIC

Ingredients

- 2 cups of Brussels sprouts

- 3-5 cloves of garlic

- 1 Tbsp avocado oil

- salt + pepper to taste

Instructions

1. Preheat oven to 400° F.

2. Wash and dry the sprouts.

3. Cut in half and loose outer leaves.

4. Place them directly on a baking sheet.

5. Cut the garlic cloves and cut into large pieces.

6. Mix the sprouts and garlic with avocado oil, salt, and pepper.

7. Bake for 15 min, then stir sprouts and garlic.

8. Cook another 15 to 20 min (the total cooking time depends on the size of your sprouts).

Prep time: 7 min; **Servings:** 2

Macros: Cal 106 | Carbs 9 g | Protein 3g | Fat 7 g Saturated Fat 1 g Fiber 3 g | Sugar 1 g

SIMPLE VEGAN BOK CHOY SOUP

Ingredients

- 2 chopped bok choy stalks

- 1 cup vegetable broth

- 1 tsp nutritional yeast

- 2 dashes of garlic powder

- 2 pinches of onion powder

- salt and pepper to taste

Instructions

1. Mix all ingredients in a bowl and mix.

2. Microwave for 3 min

Prep time: 1 min; **Servings:** 1

Macros: Sodium 205 mg Carbs 4 g Fiber 1 g Sugar 2 g

BAKED TOFU FRIES

Ingredients

- 15.5 g of extra tofu firmly drained and squeezed

- 2 Tbsp olive oil

- ½ tsp basil

- ½ tsp oregano

- ¼ tsp pepper

- ¼ tsp cayenne pepper

- ¼ tsp onion powder

- ¼ tsp garlic powder

- Salt and pepper

Instructions

1. Preheat the oven to 375° F.

2. Mix the olive oil and all the herbs and spices.

3. Cut tofu into long strips about ¼ - ½ "thick and cover with marinade.

4. Place the strips on a parchment paper and cook for 20 min. Turn and bake another 15-20 min, or until crispy on the outside.

Prep time:30 min; **Servings:** 4

Macros: Cal 132 | Carbs 3g | Protein 7g | Fat 10 g Saturated Fat 1 g | Cholesterol 0 mg | Sodium 40 mg Potassium 213 mg | Fiber 0 g | Sugar 1 g | Vitamin A: 115 IU | Calcium: 39 mg | Iron: 1.2 mg

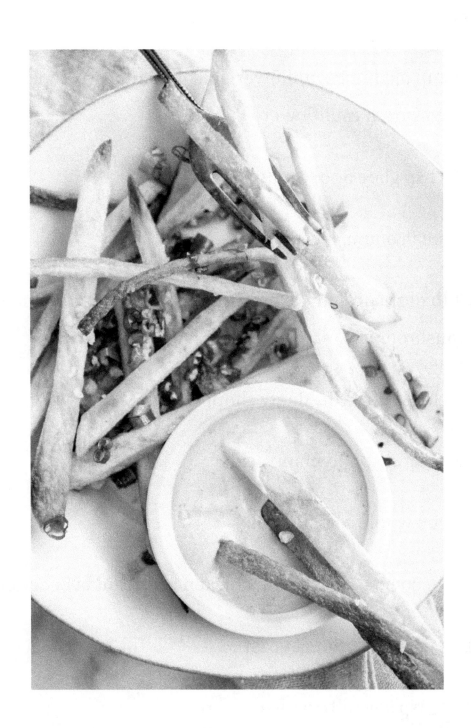

CAULIFLOWER MUSHROOM RISOTTO

Ingredients

3. 1 cup medium cauliflower gold 4-5 cups pre-cooked fresh gold frozen cauliflower

4. 1 Tbsp ghee or coconut oil

5. 1 small onion, diced

6. 1 lb of small shiitake mushrooms, sliced or cremini or white mushrooms

7. 3 cloves of garlic, finely chopped

8. 2 Tbsp coconut amino acids

9. 1 cup whole coconut milk

10. 1 cup bone broth gold chicken broth gold vegetable broth

11. ¼ cup nutritional yeast

12. ½ tsp sea salt, to taste

13. 2 Tbsp tapioca starch

14. Ground black pepper to taste (skip for AIP)

15. Chopped parsley to garnish

Instructions

1. Remove the cauliflower leaves and cut the flowers off the roots.

2. Use a cheese grater or food processor with a rasp accessory and grate the cauliflower to the size of the rice.

3. Add the butter or coconut oil in the instant saucepan and set it to "Sautéed." Cool for 5 min and cover the bottom of the pan.

4. Add the onion, mushrooms and garlic and cook, stirring, for 7 min, until the mushrooms are sweaty and soft.

5. Add the coconut amino acids and sauté 5 min until the vegetables are brown. Turn off the instant pot.

6. Add the cauliflower rice, coconut milk, bone broth, nutritional yeast, and sea salt. Stir together.

7. Close the lid, make sure the valve is closed and set the instant pot to "Manual" for 2 min

8. Release the pressure valve and open the lid.

9. Sprinkle tapioca starch on risotto and stir until thickened. Add more salt if you wish. Add ground black pepper if you use it.

10. Sprinkle with chopped parsley .

Prep time: 5 min; **Servings:** 4

Macros: Cal 299.05 Fat 19.15g Saturated Fat 15.12g Cholesterol 9.6mg Sodium 546.4mg Potassium 1036.52mg Carbs 27.61g Fiber 8.31g Sugar 8.64g Protein 10.62g

SILKY VEGAN CAULIFLOWER SOUP

Ingredients

- 1 small cauliflower gold ½ large cauliflower about 500 g gold 1 lb

- 1 Tbsp olive oil

- 2 cloves of garlic, finely chopped

- 2 sprigs of thyme

- 350 ml or 1 ½ cups of vegetable broth or water

- 120 ml or ½ cups of light coconut milk

- salt and freshly ground black pepper to taste

- 4 Tbsp pomegranate seeds to decorate

- 2 sprigs of thyme to decorate

Instructions

4. Divide the head of cauliflower into florets or cut it more or less. You can use the leaves if you want, but these will change the color of the soup.

5. Fry the chopped garlic in olive oil in a large frying pan until fragrant, about 2 min Add vegetable stock or water, sprigs of thyme and cauliflower flowers. Bring to the boil, cover, reduce heat, and cook for 15-20 min, until the cauliflower is beautiful and!

6. Discard the thyme and mix until smooth with a hand blender or food processor. You may want to work in batches.

7. Add light coconut milk and season with salt and freshly ground black pepper. Garnish with pomegranate seeds and fresh thyme.

Prep time: 10 min; **Servings:** 2

Macros: Cal 184 | Carbs 17 g | Protein 3g | Fat 11 g Saturated Fat 5 g | Sodium 791 mg | Potassium 466 mg Fiber 3g | Sugar 8 g | Vitamin A: 420 IU | Vitamin C: 69.5 mg | Calcium: 35 mg | Iron: 0.7 mg

VEGETARIAN RED CURRY STIR FRY

Ingredients

Sauce:

- 1 inch (2.5 cm) fresh ginger

- ½ tsp cumin

- ½ tsp coriander

- 2 Tbsp + 2 tsp red curry paste

- 1 cup or 235 ml full coconut milk

Baked:

5. 1 Tbsp coconut oil

6. 1 lb gold sweet potatoes

7. 1 red pepper

8. 1 medium sweet onion

9. 2 cloves of garlic

10. 5 oz sugar peas

11. fresh coriander to decorate

12. cauliflower rice to serve

Instructions

1. Grate the ginger in a small bowl using a Microplane zester. Add cumin, cilantro, and red curry paste. Stir, then add coconut and beat until well combined. Put aside.

2. Peel the sweet potatoes and cut into large cubes. Cut the peppers, onions, and garlic and set aside.

3. Heat coconut oil in a large wok or deep pan over medium heat. Add sweet potatoes to the pan and stir to cover. Bake until soft, about 8-10 min.

4. Reduce the heat to medium and add the diced bell pepper and onion to the pan. Cook for another 5 min, stirring regularly.

5. Put the peas and garlic in the pan. Bake for another 3-5 min with continuous stirring until they are sweet and crispy.

6. Remove the pan from the heat and pour the sauce into the pan. Mix to cover the vegetables, extinguish the pan with the sauce. Wait 2-3 min for the sauce to thicken and then serve cauliflower rice (see previous comments)! Top with chopped fresh coriander.

Prep time: 10 min; **Servings:** 4

Macros: Cal 88 Carbs 14g Fat 4g Protein 3g

CREAMY CAULIFLOWER GARLIC RICE

Ingredients

- 6 to 8 cups of chopped cauliflower

- 4 cups vegetable broth + 2 cups water

- ½ cup milk

- 1 ½ cups brown rice (I used a mixture of brown rice)

- 1 tsp salt (and more to taste!)

- 2 tsp

- 6-8 cloves minced garlic

- ½ cup cheese mozzarella to cover (more to taste)

Instructions

1. Cook the rice according to the instructions on the package. Put aside.

2. Cook the vegetable broth and water in a large saucepan. Add the cauliflower and cook for about 10 min, until tender. Transfer the cauliflower pieces to a blender or food processor.

3. Puree cauliflower, add extra milk or vegetable broth to a smooth, creamy consistency. Season with salt. For over cooked rice and stir to combine.

4. In a large nonstick skillet, melt butter and add garlic, and cook on low heat until very fragrant for about 3 to 5 min Add the creamy rice mixture and stir until the butter and garlic are absorbed. Add cheese or mix all the ice to melt. Season with additional salt and pepper.

Servings: 6; **Prep time:** 15 min

Macros: Cal 190 Carbs 23g Fat 9g Protein 5g

HEALTHY CAULIFLOWER FRIED RICE

Ingredients

- 1 chopped cauliflower in florets

- 1 small yellow onion, finely chopped

- ½ cup frozen peas

- ½ cup carrots, diced

- 2 beaten eggs

- 1 Tbsp sesame oil

- ¼ cup low sodium soy sauce

- 1 Tbsp light brown sugar

- ⅛ tsp ground ginger

- 1 pinch of red pepper flakes

- 2 Tbsp chopped green onion

Instructions

1. Chop the cauliflower head into florets and place in a food processor. Press until it starts to look like rice; put aside.

2. A large wok (or skillet) over medium heat and sprinkle with sesame oil. Add the onion, peas, and carrots and cook until tender, about 2 min

3. Meanwhile, mix soy sauce, brown sugar, ginger, and red pepper flakes in a small bowl; set aside.

4. Move the vegetable mixture to the side of the wok and add the beaten egg, stir until they are thoroughly cooked, then add them to the vegetables.

5. Add the cauliflower "rice" and over the soy sauce, mix well. Cook another 3 to 4 min until cauliflower is tender and soft.

6. Top with green onions.

Prep time: 10 min; **Servings:** 4

Macros: Cal 131 Fat 6.3 g Saturated Fat 1.3 g Carbs 13.5 g Fiber 3 g Protein 6.5 g Sugar 7.1 g

MEXICAN CAULIFLOWER RICE BURRITO BOWL

Ingredients

- 3-3 ½ cups of cauliflower rice

- 1 Tbsp olive oil

- ½ chopped red onion

- 2 garlic cloves, finely chopped

- ½ tsp garlic powder

- 1 tsp cumin

- ½ tsp oregano

- pinch of cayenne pepper

- salt and pepper to taste

- 1 can of black beans 11-14 oz

- 1 diced tomato

- Sliced avocado

- Slices of lemons

- handful of coriander

Instructions

For cauliflower rice:

1. Break the cauliflower into florets and place it in a food processor.

2. The cauliflower pulse is similar to rice. Remove and place on a clean towel or paper towels and wring out any excess liquid.

3. Meanwhile, heat oil over medium heat and add onion and garlic. Saute 2 to 3 min until fragrant and transparent.

4. Add cauliflower, garlic powder, cumin, oregano, cayenne pepper and salt and pepper to taste.

5. Continue cooking regularly, stir for another 8 to 10 min

Bowl assembly:

1. Add Mexican cauliflower

2. black beans, drained and rinsed

3. chopped tomato and chopped red onion remaining

4. slices of avocado

5. sprinkle with lime juice

Prep time:10 min **Servings:** 2-3

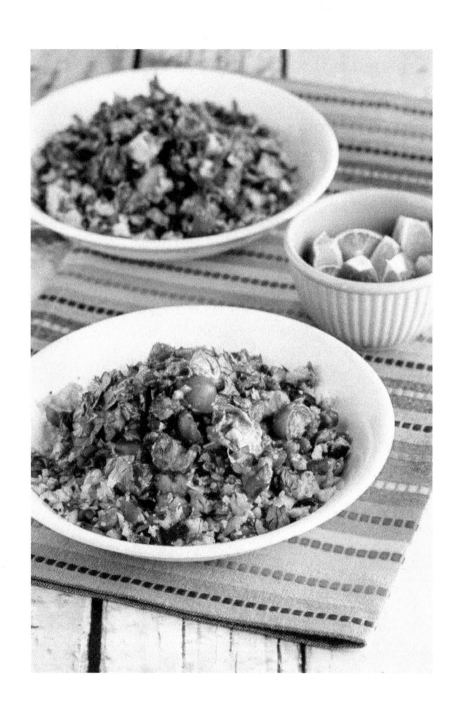

CAULIFLOWER FIESTA RICE SALAD

Ingredients

Salad:

- 1 small cauliflower

- ¼ cup finely chopped red onion

- cup corn

- ½ cup black beans

- 3 jalapeños, finely chopped, without seeds or ribs

- 1 packet (10 g) of tomatoes, grapes or cherries, cut in half

- ⅓ cup fresh cheese or cheese cotija (feta also works)

- ⅓ cup chopped fresh coriander

Bandage:

- 2 lime juice

- 1 orange juice

- 1 Tbsp olive oil

- ½ tsp chili powder

- ¼ tsp cumin

- 1 small clove of garlic

Instructions

1. Prepare the cauliflower rice: cut the cauliflower into large florets. Place the ⅓ of the florets in a food processor. Press until the cauliflower looks like grains of rice. Place the cauliflower rice in a large bowl. Repeat this process 2 more times with the florets.

2. Prepare the salad: add the onion, corn, black beans, jalapeno, tomatoes, cheese, and coriander to the cauliflower rice bowl.

3. Prepare the vinaigrette: add all the ingredients of the vinaigrette to the food processor or blender. Mix until smooth. For salad dressing over salad and mix to combine.

Prep time: 20 min; **Servings:** 8

Macros: Cal 284 Fat 25.6 g Carbohydrate 8.8 g Fiber 3.6 g Sugar 2.2 g Protein 5.8 g Net Carbohydrate 5 g

CURRIED CAULIFLOWER RICE KALE SOUP

Ingredients

- 5-6 cups of cauliflower flowers

- 2 to 3 Tbsp curry powder or curry powder

- 1 tsp garlic powder

- ½ tsp cumin

- ½ tsp sweet pepper

- ¼ tsp sea salt

- 2-3 Tbsp olive oil for frying

- 3/4 cup chopped red onion

- 1 tsp minced garlic

- 2 tsp olive oil or avocado

- 8 kale leaves with the stems removed and chopped

- 2 cups (5 oz) chopped carrots

- 4 cups broth

- 1 cup almond milk or coconut milk

- ½ tsp red gold pepper chili flakes

- ½ tsp black pepper

- Salt after cooking

Instructions

1. Preheat the oven to 400° F.

2. Mix the cauliflower flowers in a small bowl with curry powder, garlic powder, cumin, pepper, salt, and 3 Tbsp oil.

3. Spread cauliflower flowers in a baking dish or on a roasting pan. Place in the oven and cook for 20 to 22 min, but without boiling. Something not cooked.

4. While the cauliflower cools, prepare the remaining vegetables on a chopping board.

5. Then place the bouquets of cauliflower in a food processor or press several times until cauliflower is chopped or "chopped." See the picture in the publication.

6. Once in a while, prepare your pot.

7. Place the onion, 2 tsp oil, and chopped garlic in a large saucepan. Bake for 5 min until fragrant.

8. Then add broth, milk, vegetables, cauliflower "rice" and red pepper and black pepper.

9. Bring it to a boil (make sure the milk does not overheat) and simmer another 20 min until the vegetables are well cooked.

10. If necessary, add a pinch of sea salt when ready to serve.

11. Garnish with herbs and crumble the nuts/cookies with the seeds.

Prep time: 30 min; **Servings:** 4

Macros: Cal 162 Sugar 6 g Sodium 250 mg Fat 8 g Saturated Fat 1.3 g Carbs 20 g Fiber 9 g Protein 6 g

PESTO CAULIFLOWER RICE

Ingredients

- 3 cups of cauliflower rice (see note)

- 1 Tbsp olive oil

- 2 cups shredded kale stalks

- ⅓ to ½ cup extra virgin olive oil

- 1 clove of garlic

- ½ lemon juice

- ⅓ cup grated Parmesan cheese

- 3 Tbsp chopped walnuts

Instructions

1. Add the oil in a large skillet and bring to medium heat. Add the cauliflower and cook until tender.

2. Add pesto Ingredients to a food processor to make pesto. Press for a few min until it reaches a thick sauce consistency.

The pesto will be ready to be very thick, but it will be a few min later. If it does not decompose, add a little more olive oil until it decomposes. Test and adjust if necessary. Depending on the type of cabbage and your personal preferences, you may want to add cheese, oil, lemon, etc.

3. Add the cauliflower rice pesto. Start with a few Tbsp and add if necessary until you have the desired taste. You may not need the full amount, and you can not use the pesto for another .

4. Serve hot cauliflower rice. Garnish with more Parmesan if desired.

Prep time: 10 min; **Servings:** 4

Macros: Cal 293 Fat 26.6 g Carbohydrate 8.8 g Fiber 3.6 g Sugar 2.2 g Protein 5.8 g Net Carbohydrate 5 g

BLISSFUL BASIL SWEET POTATOES

Ingredients

For roasted sweet potatoes:

6. 4 cups sweet potatoes, peeled and cut into 1-inch cubes

7. 2 Tbsp grapeseed oil or other heat-tolerant oil

8. 1 Tbsp ground cinnamon

9. 1 Tbsp smoked pepper

10. fine-grained sea salt

11. For the spicy cauliflower rice

12. 1 head of about 6 heartless cups cauliflower and cut into bouquets

13. 1 Tbsp sesame oil

14. 5 onions, sliced and thinly sliced

15. 1 cup cherry tomatoes or grapes in wedges

16. 2-3 Tbsp apple cider vinegar or rice vinegar

17. 1-2 Tbsp reduced-sodium Tamari *

18. 1-2 Tbsp garlic and chili paste or Sriracha

19. Cup chopped chives

20. ¼ cup chopped fresh cilantro

21. For the smashed avocado

22. 1 ripe avocado cut in half, pitted and peeled

23. 1 Tbsp fresh lime juice 1 garlic clove, chopped to taste

24. Sea salt to taste

Instructions

For roasted sweet potatoes:

1. Preheat the oven to 425 ° F. Cover a large baking sheet with parchment paper.

2. Place the sweet potatoes on a baking sheet, sprinkle with oil, and sprinkle with cinnamon, pepper, and sea salt to taste. Mix to cover.

3. Roast for 25 to 30 min or until soft and return every 15 min

4. For the spicy cauliflower rice

5. Add the cauliflower florets to the bowl of a food processor equipped with an S knife. Press to finely chop the size of the rice kernels.

6. Heat the sesame oil in a large wok gold fry over medium heat. Add the cauliflower, chives, and tomatoes and cook for 8 to 10 min or until the cauliflower softens, stirring occasionally.

7. Mix apple cider vinegar, tamari, and chili and garlic paste in a small bowl. For the sauce over the cauliflower and cook another 6 to 8 min, or until the "rice" turns into light golden color and the liquid is absorbed, stirring regularly. Remove from heat and add the onions and cilantro.

For the smashed avocado:

1. Use the back of a fork in a small bowl to mix the avocado, juice lime, garlic, and sea salt.

2. Place the sweet potatoes and cauliflower in bowls, squeeze them together, cover with a generous spoonful of mashed avocado.

Prep time: 15 min; **Servings:** 3

Macros: Cal 605 | Carbs 100 g | Protein 13 g | Fat 22 g | Fiber: 23 g | Sugar 22 g |

SUSHI VEGAN CAULIFLOWER RICE

Ingredients

- 4 sheets of nori

- 2 cups of cauliflower rice

- 1 red pepper sliced thinly

- 1 avocado, peeled and sliced

- 1 cup finely sliced red cabbage

- 2 green onions sliced all over

- 2 cups of chopped field vegetables

- Peanut sauce

- ¼ cup peanut butter

- 1 tsp stevia

- 2 tsp tamari or Bragg

- 1 tsp Sriracha according to your heat preference

- 2 tsp chopped peanuts to cover

Instructions

1. Place a sheet of nori on a bamboo roll. Cover half a thin layer of cauliflower rice. With thin slices of red pepper, avocado slices, sliced red cabbage, green onion slices, and some field vegetables.

2. Use the bamboo roll with your finger. Roll it firmly to the end.

3. Prepare the sauce by combining peanut butter, agave, Bragg (or tamari), and sriracha. Stir to combine. Add 1 to 3 tsp water to obtain good immersion. Sprinkle top with chopped peanuts.

4. Cut the roll into 5 to 6 cm.

Prep time: 10 min; **Servings:** 8

Macros: Cal 73, Carbs 14g, Fat 5g Protein 9g

SPANISH CAULIFLOWER RICE

Ingredients

- 2 Tbsp avocado oil (or olive oil)

- ½ cup chopped white onion

- 1 lb of cauliflower (about 3 cups)

- 1 cup vegetable broth

- 1 cup enchilada sauce

- garlic salt, chili powder, cumin (optional spices, see comments)

- lime juice (optional)

- coriander (optional, to decorate)

Instructions

1. Heat the oil in a saucepan over high heat. Add chopped onion and stir for 1 minute until it is transparent.

2. Add the curry cauliflower and the vegetable broth. Boil again and stir for a few min

3. Add the sauce enchilada, reduce the heat and cover. Simmer 15-20 min until most liquids are absorbed.

4. Squeeze the lime juice and the selection of herbs and cover with coriander.

Prep time:5 min; **Servings:** 4

Macros: Cal 73, Carbs 14g, Fat 5g Protein 9g

FRITTERS WITH CHIPOTLE LIME AIOLI

Ingredients

- 1 cup organic cauliflower without leaves (looking for 4 cups oFresh cauliflower rice)

- 3 large eggs raised in the meadow, a little beaten

- ½ cup blanched almond flour *

- 2 Tbsp coconut flour

- 1 tsp of baking powder (aspect without aluminum and corn)

- 1 tsp garlic powder

- ½ tsp chipotle powder (use chili powder or smoked paprika for less heat or book)

- ½ tsp sea salt (plus sea salt extra flakes to serve)

- freshly ground black pepper

- 2 to 4 Tbsp butter, olive oil, coconut oil, avocado oil or other cooking oil

- ½ cup homemade mayonnaise or avocado oil mayonnaise purchased in-store

- ½ tsp chipotle powder

- 1 tsp fresh lime juice

- ½ tsp fresh grated lime

- ⅛ tsp garlic powder

Instructions

1. Remove the green leaves from the head of the cauliflower. Cut the cauliflower head into small florets, remove the kernel and discard. Wash the florets until they are dehydrated. You can also dry with paper towels. You do not want to be wet at all.

2. Add the florets to your food processor. Press several times or process.

3. Put 4 cups fresh cauliflower rice in a large mixing bowl. Add beaten eggs, almond flour, coconut flour, baking powder, garlic powder, chipotle powder, salt, and pepper. Mix well and let stand about 10 min Most of the liquid is absorbed, if

there is a lot of liquid, it is poured, or a little more coconut flour is added.

4. The heat has a frying pan or skillet. We have a tsp over medium heat. When hot, add enough oil to cover the bottom of the pan. With 2 to 4 Tbsp dough, form burgers with your hands and place them carefully in the hot pan. Work in batches and do not overload the container.

5. Bake until the bottom is brown, about 3 to 4 min, then flip gently and cook another 3 min Go to a plate with paper towels.

6. Repeat this with the remaining dough and add more if necessary.

7. In a small bowl, mix mayonnaise, chipotle, juice and lemon zest, and garlic powder.

Prep time: 15 min; **Servings:** 4

Macros: Cal 605 | Carbs 100 g | Protein 13 g | Fat 22 g | Fiber: 23 g | Sugar 22 g |

CONCLUSION

I'm so glad you've made it this far, I'm sure this journey into the world of keto meat has been amazing, have you tasted these dishes with the whole family? with friends? have you seen how quick and easy they were to prepare.

Keep practicing, keep cooking, keep trying and keep trying, you will be great!

I always recommend talking to a nutritionist before any diet or nutritional change.

Thank you and I look forward to future recipes.